The Complete Bread Machine Cookbook

A comprehensive Machine Cookbook. Learn New Simple, Easy and Delicious Bread Machine Recipes for Smart People

MEGAN NEEL

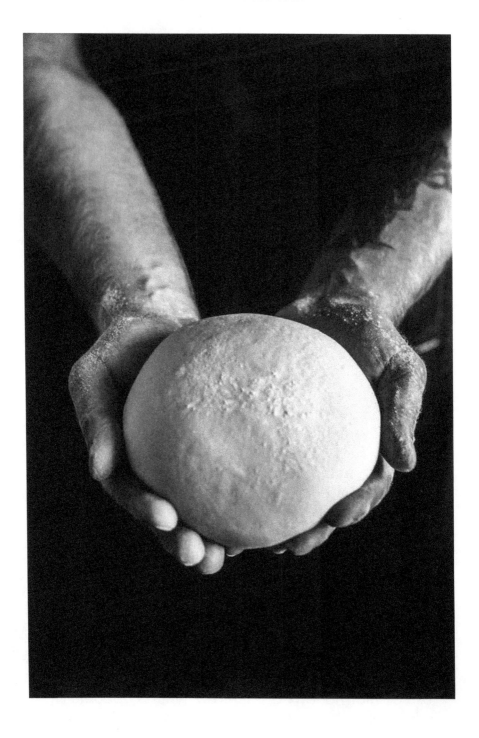

TABLE OF CONTENT

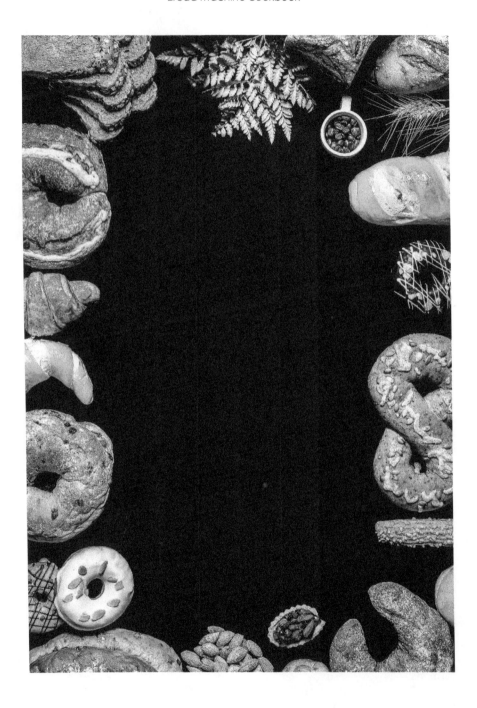

Introduction:

Matsushita Electric, which is now popularly recognized as Panasonic, launched the first bread machine in Japan in 1986. In most countries where bread is their staple meal, the bread machine was successful and was widely used in most American kitchens in the 1990s. The conventional bread-making method is laborious, and the bread machine allows the process of bread-making a quick and time-consuming process. Simply pour the ingredients needed into the unit. Simply press the button after pouring the rice, yeast, and wet ingredients. All the ingredients are combined well, and a tiny blade is kneaded, and the dough is made. The machine's internal temperature will increase automatically, and the dough will be cooked.

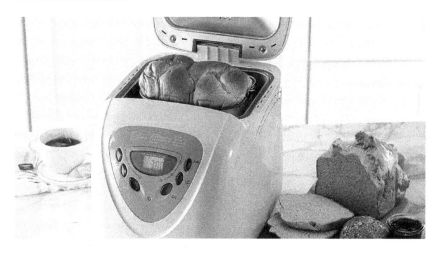

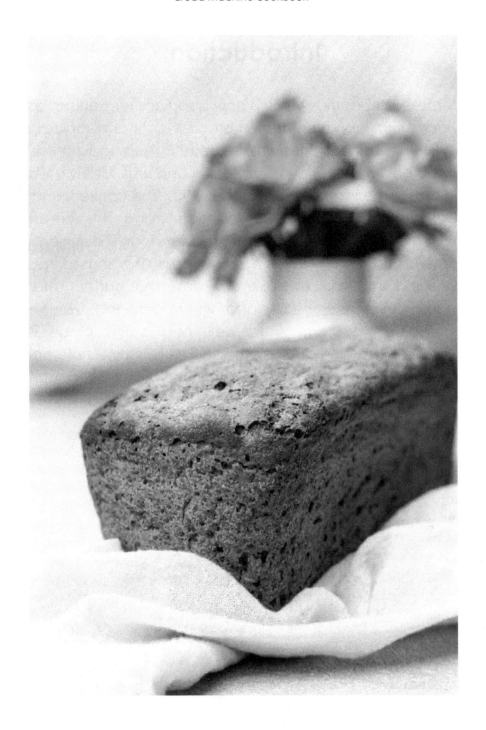

Chapter 1: Main ingredients

Measurements are not just a recommendation when it comes to baking. Instead, it is science. To weigh the ingredients, you have to be very patient. Make sure you go to a kitchen store or buy online to stock your kitchen with true measuring instruments, for instance. Be sure you've got different sizes of liquid and dry measurement equipment.

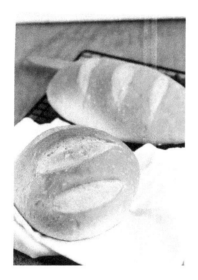

The key errors you don't want to repeat include:

Water

The liquid part used most in bread is water. It is, just as flour is, one of the important ingredients.

Milk

Milk is the second liquid substance that is used the most, aside from water—milk in order to add spice. The milk used in bread recipes must be lukewarm, just like water, particularly when combined directly with yeast.

Salt

When adding salt, you have to keep one simple law in mind; keep it away from the yeast. The salt will kill the fermentation if the sugar helps ferment the yeast.

Do not use liquid dry ingredient proportions, and vice versa,

The wet and dry teaspoons and tablespoons are interchangeable. However, cups are not. There must be two liquid cups if you like two cups of water. Don't you think there's any difference? Using a scale for a dry cup and fill it with sweat. Then, pipe it into your mixing cup of liquid. Quickly, you can find that the calculation is less than precise.

Flour

White flour is one of the kitchen's most commonly used products; it is undoubtedly one of the most common bistro meds. Only think about how it is mentioned in almost all recipes: the generic word "flour" does not imply completely Zero if used alone. It'd be like suggesting you have to use meat to prepare a decent broth: yeah, but which one? You're going to create a good broth with beef fillets! Great beef, for goodness sake, but totally unacceptable for any lengthy cooking. The same happens to flours: for example, the most ideal for a long-leavening recipe - a brioche - is completely unacceptable for the preparation of short crust pastry. It will be much easier to discern the most acceptable form of flour for the preparation - thus, for those who compose the recipes.

The form of wheat from which they are derived relies on the first difference between the two varieties of flour: soft wheat and durum wheat. Durum wheat flours are strongly yellowish, grainier to the touch, and are used mostly for the preparation of pasta and some forms of bread. The description of 'durum wheat semolina' or 'durum wheat flour' is also seen on offer. On the other side, the soft wheat ones are white in color, have a quality of almost "dusty," and are definitely the most used in confectionery and bread baking. They often vary based on the wheat from which they are obtained: the United States, Canada, and Argentina are the countries with the strongest soft grains, such as Manitoba, Plata. Uh, among some.

Enzymes, sugars, proteins, mineral salts are the most important substances which make up flour - restricting the topic to its use in cooking. In baking, enzymes are definitely the substances that play the fundamental function. These are separated into protease and amylase. The former targets the flour starch and creates the basic yeast food. On the other side, the latter attacks the gluten, making it more elastic. The sugars are used, allowing them to expand and develop to feed the yeast. Two forms are the essential proteins: soluble and insoluble. Gliadin and glutenin are the most significant, always inside a culinary discourse.

Throughout the dough, these proteins bind together to form GLUTEN. It should also be pointed out in this respect that there is another indicator: the W value, which is used to mean the 'power' of the flour.

In comparison to the following results, poor flour and 'power' flour are categorized as flour in the following categories:

- Weak - up to 170 W. Cookie flour, waffles, breadsticks, and little pastries. In water, they consume approximately 50 percent of their weight.

- Intermediate-180 to 260 W. Leavened dough flour that needs an average quantity of water (or other liquids), such as French bread, oil, or some forms of pizza. They consume 55%-65% of their water weight and are the most frequently used in pizzerias.

- 280 to 350 W powerful. Flours that need a significant volume of water (or other liquids) such as baba, brioches, naturally leavened pastries, and pizza with leavened dough are useful in making bread. They consume about 65 percent of their weight in water, 75 percent of it.

Types of Flour

Soft wheat flour: flour obtained from the milling of soft wheat, with thin, round granules, is the most frequently used in the bread-making method and, according to the rule, is the only flour that may be put on the market under the name 'flour,' accompanied by the form which, depending on the fiber and protein content, is defined by the following numbers: 00 (double zero), 0,1,2 and whole meal. The 00 separates the whiter flour, but also the lowest in fiber and protein, which, along with the 0, is most often used in the preparation of bakery goods, not only domestic but also artisanal and agricultural.

-Manitoba flour: this kind of flour, distinguished by a high content of gliadins and glutenin's, proteins responsible for the production of gluten, has spread with some success in recent years, as already described. A special form of soft wheat seed produced predominantly in an area of Canada (Manitoba), originally populated by indigenous peoples, is obtained by milling Manitoba grain. The value of Manitoba flour is that it achieves a rather exuberant leavening mechanism maintained by a particularly solid and lightweight gluten mesh, without undue kneading effort. The result obtained would be a particularly light and fragrant bread until baked; nevertheless, the bread will become very rubbery after a few hours and not quite capable of preservation. Manitoba is ideal for doughs, which are especially rich in sugar and fat and therefore need a particularly long leavening period (panettone, baba, etc.).

-The flours of form 1 and 2 are less precious and widespread; nevertheless, they are wheat flours which are obtained with a less refined degree of milling. Generally speaking, in Northern European countries, they are very widespread and, while they are obtained by milling wheat, they help to prevent the unnecessary leavening of some forms of bread, provided their greater weight.

-The highest fiber content and outstanding nutritious value of whole meal flour, although its presence is the least appealing, particularly for us Mediterranean's.

- -Rye flour, second only to wheat, is widely used in the production of bread, especially in the German-speaking countries of Europe but also in northern Italy and South Tyrol. There are two types: a summer one and a winter one that tends to have stronger characteristics for baking. Rye grain, heavier than the wheat flour in which it is typically blended, provides a very distinctive color and fragrance to baking products. The gluten content is rather close to that of wheat, which allows for a bread that is very soft and very tasty.

-In order to produce polenta, corn flour is required. In certain nations, such as Mexico, it makes the cooking of regular tortillas, regarded in the same way as wheat, while essential substances such as calcium and some vitamins are totally absent. If we ever choose to use corn flour for the baking of any items, because of the modest amount of gluten present, we would have to pick a flour with a rather fine grain and combine it with at least 45/50 percent wheat flour.

-Oat flour is high in nutrition and minerals, but since it does not produce gluten-forming proteins, it must be combined with wheat flour to the following extent: 25% of oat flour and 75% of wheat or rye flour around bread-making. To achieve a lighter bread, it is also necessary to use oat flakes, thus retaining the proportions mentioned above.

- Millet flour in Asia and Africa is especially widespread. Although flour enriches the flavor of food, it cannot be used alone for the manufacture of bread but must also be combined with outstanding quality wheat flour in the following proportions: 20% millet flour and 80% wheat flour.

-Potato flour is very close to wheat flour for nutritional quality; adding some (20 percent) to wheat flour gives it taste, softness and improves leavening.

-Rice flour is the richest cereal in absolute starch and can be used in bread making, but it must be combined with especially strong wheat flour because of its absolute lack of proteins that enable gluten to shape (10 percent and 90 percent wheat flour).

-Buckwheat flour is primarily used for the preparation of traditional dishes such as pizzoccheri, and 10/15 percent combined with wheat flour may also be used for bread baking. It gives an unusually dark color and a slightly bitter taste to the bread.

About The Yeast

VARIOUS TYPES OF YEAST

Yeasts are classified as all substances that lead to an increase in the volume after fermentation of the dough.

Yeast for beer. This form of yeast is usually used for home baking and was historically derived from the beer must fermentation residues, although today it is produced from molasses, a by-product of the production of beet and sugar cane, and compressed and sold in 25-gram home baking cakes and 500-gram skilled baking cakes. The 25-gram bread is inferred as the comparison is made to 'panetto' in the recipes. However, beware that this is not a statute!

Brewer's yeast may also be dried in granules, typically in sachets with a dosage of 500 grams of flour.

Natural Yeast or Yeast Mother. It is suitable for producing some forms of bread and certain bread cakes (doves, panettone, etc.) and is obtained by sustained fermentation of wheat, water, also with the addition of some fermentation-promoting agents such as yogurt, raw honey, or quite ripe berries. Usually, according to the different recipes, the fermented dough is subjected to a process of refreshments and/or cleaning.

Chapter 2: Storing tips

It's pretty simple to store your bread, and it can be accomplished when you make your bread. Store the products in the freezer or anywhere in your refrigerator.

Prior to freezing, sandwich loaves can be cut. In your refrigerator, you should only just pull out what you can use and save the remainder for later. If you intend to freeze the bread, it is really necessary to cool the loaves after baking to ensure that it has finished the cooldown period. Remove all the unnecessary air by cutting and applying it to the freezer bags.

You can bake more than you, your colleagues, and your friends can consume in one sitting. Bread machine bread is so tasty. Here are few ideas for preserving creations for your bread machine:

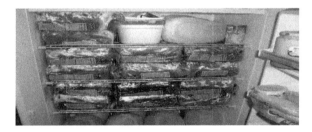

Dough. Take the dough out from the system during the kneading period. You should store it in the refrigerator if you intend on using the dough within 3 days. Shape the dough into a disk and put it in a sealable freezer bag or store the dough in a plastic wrap-covered, lightly oiled tub. In the oven, the yeast activity would not end, so punch the dough down until it's completely chilled, and then once a day. Take the dough from the refrigerator until you are about to bake bread, shape it, let it grow, and bake. There are no preservatives in the bread machine dough, so ice it if you can't bake it in three days. Shape the dough into a disk and put it in a freezer bag that is sealable. For up to a month, you can freeze bread dough. Take the dough from the freezer until you are about to bake the bread, store it overnight in the refrigerator, form it, let it grow, and bake. Until refrigerating or freezing, you may mold the dough into braids, loaves, knots, or other forms. Tightly seal the shapes and stack them in the refrigerator or freezer (if you are baking within 24 hours). Unwrap the dough at the proper moment, cause it to rise at room temperature, and bake it.

As long as commercially produced assortments are concerned, try not to accept the handmade bread can stay. Newly cooked bread is definitely not going to go long at any rate in our kitchen.

So, when it's fully cooled down, I store it in the kitchen in a bread canister.

Specialists maintain that covering it tightly in foil or locking it in a plastic pack and holding it at room temperature is the best solution to preserving bread. On the premise that staling is normally quick at regular cooler temperatures, the tendency to refrigerate bread is continually resisted.

Now that all this delicious homemade bread is in your hands, how do you store it to keep it fresh? Believe it or not, the safest choice is to ice your bread. Bread can be kept in a freezer for up to 2 months and warned if required. If you intend to consume your bread immediately after baking, one way to go is to keep it uncovered. The inside should be perfect, even though the crust gets a little rough.

Storing it in a bread box is an old-fashioned way to carry bread around longer. The bread is then wrapped and not open to the air. To protect the bread may even be wrapped in plastic, only make sure it is put with no moisture in a cold, dry location. Do not bring fresh bread in the freezer, whatever you intend to do, so it would dry out.

We don't want to waste any single slice of bread we've made; we want to share it with others, and we want to have it till supper. So, don't let your bread go out of freshness, shop bread correctly, obey the instructions at all times. You love baking.

Storage of the Remaining Bread

Bread storage isn't always convenient. You can know the right places to preserve them so that you can keep them healthy longer if you manage not to consume any of the tasty sweets that you bake. When it comes to preserving bread, there are lots of different items to bear in mind, but homemade bread is extremely fragile. To help you get the best out of your storage, here are some tips:

Don't stock a refrigerator of bread. Although this may sound like the answer to freshness, it simply affects the starch molecules' orientation, which is what allows the bread to go stale. Hold it on the counter or in the bread box whether you have leftovers from what you have cooked.

Making sure you don't let your bread hang around for too long. You have a small period of time to roll it up and protect the freshness inside until you break it into a loaf. If the interior is exposed to the environment for so long, it can tend to harden even faster and grow stale.

Do not place it in a plastic bag if your house or the bread itself is wet. The heating will promote condensation, which in the humid, moist atmosphere will prompt mold formation. Before storing it, wait until the bread cools fully.

Pre-sliced and store-bought bread can go bad even sooner, mainly because of both the ingredients and exposure (which, ironically, are sometimes to retain freshness). If you use your bread machine for baking your own bread, and you manage to have leftovers, these tips will ensure you get the best out of your bread.

Moisture Matters

The humidity and moisture in your home can control the longevity of your bread, much as with the baking phase. It would also impact the choices for storage that you have. You could leave bread on the counter overnight if the weather is more humid. As a consequence, though, it could have a thinner crust. Too much humidity ensures that before storage, you need to put your bread in airtight containers to extract as much air and humidity as you can.

That implies enabling the bread to cool to room temperature before placing it into containers or plastic bags. When it first comes out of the bread machine, you may still want to hold off on slicing the bread. If you are trying to consume the whole loaf in a limited amount of time, waiting is the safest plan. Steam falls out as you break it into warm bread. The vapor is moisture, which helps to hold the bread healthy and tasty. You'll miss the freshness if you cut off too fast.

If you leave bread on the counter because it's too dry, it'll turn into a brick easily. For fresh bread, the shortage of humidity is too much, and for most store-bought types, even too much. Humidity is a balance, and in your kitchen, you have to figure out what works with your bread. Note that it can usually last for longer than light sandwich bread, French bread, whole grain bread, and other hard bread.

If you store your bread in plastic too rapidly or too long, as we described before, the crust would become soft. You may prevent this, though, by leaving the bread on the counter or lightly covering it with a cloth or paper until it's cold. This is important for crust-lovers. It's just about finding out what fits and preferences in your house, so feel free to explore storage options, too.

To Freeze or Not to Freeze?

You can freeze your bread. You simply need to be confident, however, that you are doing things the correct way. First of all, to better collect and hold moisture, make sure the bread is cooled at ambient temperature and that you have paper or fabric wrapped around it. Seal or firmly wrap it tightly and store it away for up to six months. A vacuum sealer is preferably used to guarantee that the bread is completely packed.

Actually, the challenge in freezing bread and other baked products is not in the freezing process but in the thawing process. It is crucial that you take the bread out of the freezer in advance. You ought to let it thaw out instead of defrosting it in the refrigerator or oven. This would make it easier for the bread to re-absorb any moisture lost during the freezing process, keeping it healthy and tasty. You should throw it in the oven for a couple of minutes to cook it up until the bread gets to room temperature.

It is tricky to reheat bread. In reheating or preserving bread, moisture is the main challenge, and freezing will impact it in several different ways. It's going to be up to you to work out the right ways for your bread to be processed and reheated, so these suggestions can hopefully help.

Other Storage Solutions

The bread box alternative still exists. For decades, many bakers have been using

them, and even if they are not as common now as they were 20 years ago, they still exist. The best option for your bread is a bread box? Consider a few things:

The package is made of storage material. Metal creates a major improvement relative to wooden crates. Based on other elements, it may also affect storage and shelf-life.

What sort of bread do you store? Both pieces of bread are distinct and, when processed, react differently. Making sure you take the time, as well as what is right for them, to get to know your bread types.

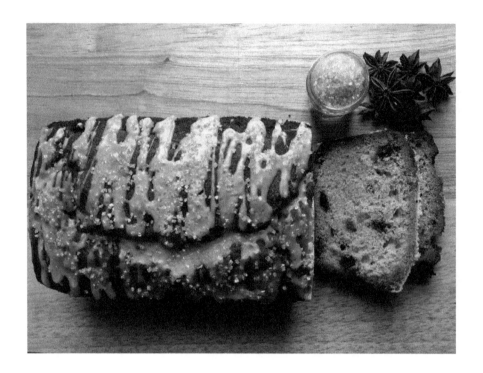

Chapter 3: Tips and tricks

This segment will provide you all sorts of useful tips to ensure that you make the most of your baking, whether you're just baking bread for the first time or you just want to bake better treats. You can find it all here, from essential elements to fast fixes and even plain fundamentals.

Don't skip the salt!

Unless you directly change a sodium content recipe (in this case, you can find a low or no-sodium version), for whatever excuse, salt is an element, and you can't leave it out. And if it looks like it's not going to make a difference, a recipe may be destroyed.

Get a conversion chart, app, or magnet for the fridge.

There are also conversion manuals for kitchens out there that you can have on file. That way, you know precisely how to do things whether you decide to convert measurements or make substitutions. When you have conversions and substitutions at hand at all times, you'll find all of your preparation and baking to be more fun.

If you're always in the early days, before you have the feel of it, you'll want to stick to the book as much as you can. You should throw these laws out of the window until you branch out and begin to explore. The deliciousness of baking is in the specifics, and when it comes to proportions, you cannot afford to make basic errors.

There is a justification for the recipe; please obey the directions to the letter if you want to get the best results.

Quality Matters

The consistency of the products that you use can make a difference while you are making something. That's not to suggest the flour from the supermarket brand is not as good as the brand name, since it could be really good. However, in order to get great outcomes, you should be vigilant in picking good quality ingredients. Go to a baker's supply or a nearby bakery shop, if you have the option, to get the nice stuff at better rates. If not, please ensure that your essential ingredients are known to you and which ones are better.

The more acquainted you are with your own baking expertise and tastes, the more you can determine where consistency counts most about yourself. Hold these tips in mind before then. Even while you're making bread, note the greater protein quality counts for your flour. More protein, which allows healthier bread, suggests stronger gluten. The smoother feel of cake flour and lower protein count render it suitable for making cakes and other sweets.

Recipes All Have a Reason

A lot of people like to simply "throw in" or weigh the ingredients fast, which is great whether you're an expert or if you're making something you've made 100 times before. If you want to recreate something from a recipe book, however, you need to adapt the recipe. You may transform your bread into something entirely different than what you wanted, including a single missing ingredient or mismeasurement.

It's not that you are going to destroy anything with careless disregard by taking up baking. If you're new to the bread machine game, however, before you throw caution to the wind and throw the formula aside once you know the baking temperature, you can get used to what you're doing.

You may want to write down at least an approximate approximation of what the measurement is, even though you prepare your own recipes over time. Recipes that don't have finite measurements are challenging to post. Although you may know precisely how much a "little" salt is, most individuals can't reliably quantify it. It requires skills to cook, but baking is a process, and it should be regarded as well.

Buttermilk Basics

Some people do not even realize precisely what buttermilk is. A ton of people doesn't realize what this strange baking ingredient is about. You don't have to be ashamed. Traditionally, buttermilk was what existed after the cream had been churned into sugar. Any of the buttermilk you see today on the shelf is cultured or processed.

Buttermilk is used because baked products are applied with a faint tang. By interacting with the baking soda in the recipe, often improves the development of the bread or pastry. A number of bread and pastry recipes include buttermilk. Not everybody, though, actually happens to hold buttermilk around. There is a remedy if you aren't in the habit of holding it around or if you intend to bake something at the last minute. A liquid measurement cup should be taken from you (one cup is fine). Insert a tablespoon of lemon juice into a measuring cup. Next, pump up to half a cup of milk. Enable it to settle down for a while, and voila, you've got some homemade buttermilk.

Try Something New

It is good to experiment. You do not want to break too far from the conventional if you're a beginner at baking bread or only beginning to master your bread machine. If you are able to make errors for the sake of accomplishment, however, experiment away! With your bread machine, as you get more skilled in baking bread, you would feel more relaxed modifying stuff and seeing everything you can do on your own.

You may try substitutions for products, such as the popular usage of applesauce in baked goods as a sweetener. You may incorporate spices to established recipes, adjust baking times and temperatures, and even use your bread machine to try to make your own perfect recipes.

Tests of Continuity

The major distinction relative to other cooking, for baking bread, is that you need to hold an eye on the consistency. In certain instances, though the good old "lightly brown" law holds, in a baking machine such as the bread machine, the quality may be very different. Make sure you capitalize on the "pause" feature and allow yourself the ability from time to time to check in on your baked goods to make sure they turn out to be their finest.

Your baking cycles don't need to be disrupted very much. One is expected to be plenty. It's a smart idea to stop to remove the paddle while you produce bread and, at the same time, inspect the bread to see how it's coming along. Not only does it make it easier for you to guarantee that the accuracy is accurate, but it also helps you to bring the paddle out until it is cooked into the bread and becomes a hassle to extract.

Mistakes When Making Bread

Your success in making bread in a bread machine can be affected by many different factors, which means a recipe that turns out a wonderful loaf one day may not produce the same loaf a week later. The bread will probably still be delicious, but it might not look exactly right. Here are some common bread-making issues: No rise

- Yeast is old or stored improperly
- Measurement of ingredients is wrong
- Flour has a low gluten content
- Too little yeast
- The temperature of ingredients is too high
- The temperature of ingredients is too low
- Too much salt
- Too much or too little sugar

Coarse texture

- Too much liquid
- Too little salt
- Too much yeast
- Fruit or vegetables too moist
- Weather too warm or humid

Crust too light

- The crust setting is too light
- Too little sugar
- The recipe size is too large for the bucket

Too much rise

- Too much yeast
- Too little salt
- Water temperature is incorrect
- The bucket is too small for the recipe size

Dense and short

- Bread doesn't rise (see No rise)
- Ingredients were added in the wrong order
- The dough is too dry; there is too much flour (not enough liquid)
- The size of the bucket is too large for the recipe
- Too much whole-grain flour or whole grains

- Too much-dried fruit

- Too many other ingredients such as vegetables, nuts, or coconut

Crust too thick

- Bread is left in the machine after the baking cycle is complete

- Flour has too little gluten

- Bread doesn't rise high enough (see No rise)

Sunken top

- Humidor warm weather

- Too much liquid in the recipe

- Liquid ingredients are too warm

- Ingredients were measured wrong

- The bread rose too far, disrupting the baking and cooling cycles

- Too much yeast

Mushroom top

- Too much yeast

- Too much water

- Ingredients are measured wrong

- Too much sugar or too many sweet ingredients

- The size of the bucket is not suitable for the recipe

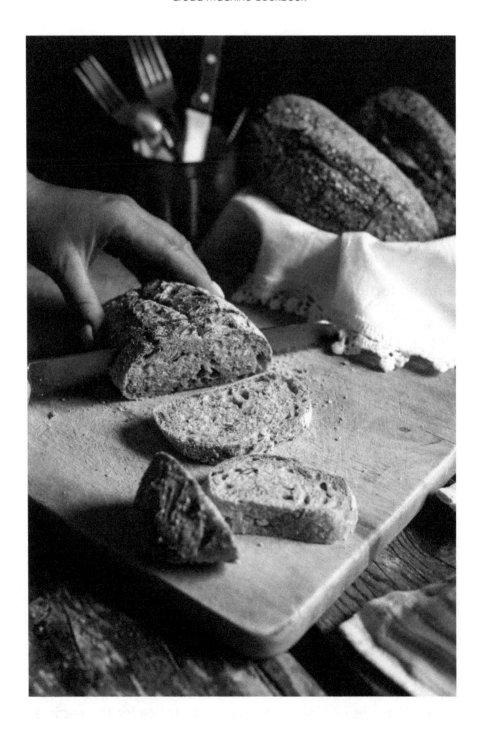

Chapter 4: Breakfast Recipes

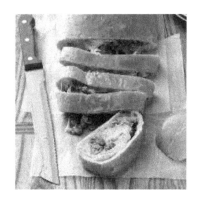

1. Chocolate Chip Scones

Preparation Time: 10 minutes

Cooking Time: 10 minutes

Servings: 8

Nutrition:

Calories: 213, Fat: 18g, Carb: 10g, Protein: 8g

Ingredients:

- 2 cups almond flour
- 1 tsp. baking soda
- ¼ tsp. sea salt
- 1 egg
- 2 Tbsp. low-carb sweetener
- 2 Tbsp. milk, cream, or yogurt
- ½ cup sugar-free chocolate chips

Directions:

- Preheat the oven to 350F.

- In a bowl, add almond flour, baking soda, and salt and blend.

- Then add the egg, sweetener, milk, and chocolate chips. Blend well.

- Pat the dough into a ball and place it on parchment paper.

- Roll the dough with a rolling pin into a large circle. Slice it into 8 triangular pieces.

- Place the scones and parchment paper on a baking sheet and separate the scones about 1 inch or so apart.

- Bake for 7 to 10 minutes or until lightly browned.

- Cool and serve.

2. Savory Waffles

Preparation Time: 10 minutes

Cooking Time: 20 minutes

Servings: 4

Nutrition:

Calories: 183, Fat: 13g, Carb: 4g, Protein: 12g

Ingredients:

- 4 eggs

- 1 tsp. olive oil

- ½ cup sliced scallions

- ¾ cup grated pepper Jack cheese

- ¼ tsp. baking soda

- 2 Pinch salt

- 1 Tbsp. coconut flour

Directions:

- Preheat the waffle iron to medium heat.

- Mix all the ingredients in a bowl. Let the batter sit for a few minutes and mix once more.

- Scoop ½ cup to 1-cup batter (depending on the waffle iron size) and pour onto the iron. Cook according to the manufacturer's directions.

- Serve warm.

3. Cheddar Biscuits

Preparation Time: 10 minutes

Cooking Time: 25 minutes

Servings: 12

Nutrition:

Calories: 125, Fat: 7g, Carb: 10g, Protein: 5g

Ingredients:

- 4 eggs
- ¼ cup unsalted butter, melted
- 1 ¼ cups, coconut milk
- ¼ tsp. salt
- ¼ tsp. baking soda
- ¼ tsp. garlic powder
- ½ cup finely shredded sharp cheddar cheese
- 1 Tbsp. fresh herb
- 2/3 cup coconut flour

Directions:

- Preheat the oven to 350F. Grease a baking sheet.
- Mix the butter, eggs, milk, salt, baking soda, garlic powder, cheese, and herbs until well blended.
- Add the coconut flour to the batter and mix until well blended. Let the batter sit for a few minutes, then mix again.

- Spoon about 2 tbsp. Batter for each biscuit onto the greased baking sheet.

- Bake for 25 minutes.

- Serve warm.

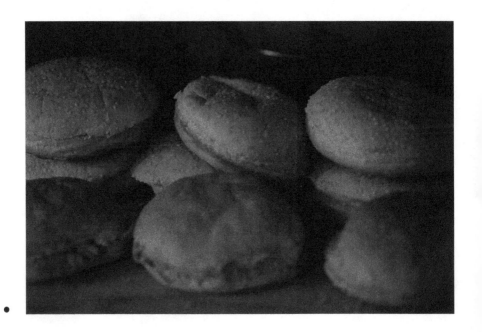

Chapter 5: Special Keto Bread Recipes

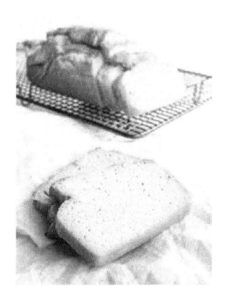

4. Sandwich Flatbread

Preparation Time: 15 minutes

Cooking Time: 20 minutes

Servings: 10

Nutrition:

Calories: 316 Fat: 6.8g Carb: 11g Protein: 25.9g

Ingredients:

- ¼ cup water
- ¼ cup oil   4 eggs
- ½ tsp. salt

- 1/3 cup unflavored whey protein powder

- ½ tsp. garlic powder

- 2 tsp. baking powder

- 6 Tbsp. coconut flour

- 3 ¼ cups almond flour

Directions:

- Preheat the oven to 325F. Combine the dry ingredients in a large bowl and mix with a hand whisk.

- Whisk in eggs, oil, and water until combined well.

- Place on a piece of large parchment paper and flatten into a rough rectangle. Place another parchment paper on top.

- Roll into a large ½ inch to ¾ inch thick rough rectangle. Transfer to the baking sheet and discard the parchment paper on top.

- Bake until it is firm to the touch, about 20 minutes.

- Cool and cut into 10 portions.

- Carefully cut each part into two halves through the bready center—stuff with your sandwich fillings.

- Serve.

5. Bread De Soul

Preparation Time: 10 minutes

Cooking Time: 45 minutes

Servings: 16

Nutrition:

Calories: 200 Fat: 15.2g Carb: 1.8g Protein: 10g

Ingredients:

- ¼ tsp. cream of tartar
- 2 ½ tsp. baking powder
- 1 tsp. xanthan gum
- 1/3 tsp. baking soda
- ½ tsp. salt
- 2/3 cup unflavored whey protein
- ¼ cup olive oil
- ¼ cup heavy whipping cream or half and half
- 2 drops of sweet leaf stevia
- 4 eggs
- ¼ cup butter
- 12 oz. softened cream cheese

Directions:

- Preheat the oven to 325F.

- In a bowl, microwave cream cheese and butter for 1 minute.

- Remove and blend well with a hand mixer.

- Add olive oil, eggs, heavy cream, and few drops of sweetener and blend well.

- Blend together the dry ingredients in a separate bowl.

- Combine the dry ingredients with the wet ingredients and mix with a spoon. Don't use a hand blender to avoid whipping it too much.

- Grease a bread pan and pour the mixture into the pan.

- Bake in the oven until golden brown, about 45 minutes.

- Cool and serve.

6. Splendid Low-Carb Bread

Preparation Time: 15 minutes

Cooking Time: 60 to 70 minutes

Servings: 12

Nutrition:

Calories: 97 Fat: 5.7g Carb: 7.5g Protein: 4.1g

Ingredients:

- ½ tsp. herbs, such as basil, rosemary, or oregano
- ½ tsp. garlic or onion powder
- 1 Tbsp. baking powder
- 5 Tbsp. psyllium husk powder
- ½ cup almond flour
- ½ cup coconut flour
- ¼ tsp. salt
- 1 ½ cup egg whites
- 3 Tbsp. oil or melted butter
- 2 Tbsp. apple cider vinegar
- 1/3 to ¾ cup hot water

Directions:

- Grease a loaf pan and preheat the oven to 350F.

- In a bowl, whisk the salt, psyllium husk powder, onion or garlic powder, coconut flour, almond flour, and baking powder.

- Stir in egg whites, oil, and apple cider vinegar. Bit by bit, add the hot water, stirring until dough increase in size. Do not add too much water.

- Mold the dough into a rectangle and transfer to a grease loaf pan.

- Bake in the oven for 60 to 70 minutes, or until crust feels firm and brown on top.

- Cool and serve.

Chapter 6: Traditional And Classic Bread Recipes

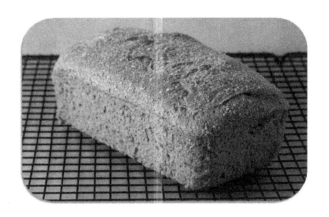

7. Irish Soda Bread

Preparation time: 10 minutes

Cooking Time: 3 hours

Servings: 16

Nutrition:

Calories 164 Fat 1.9 g Carbs 32.6 g Fiber 1.4 g Sugar 5.7 g Protein 4.3 g

Ingredients:

- 1½ cups warm water
- 2 tablespoons margarine
- 2 tablespoons white sugar
- teaspoon salt

- 4¼ cups bread flour

- tablespoons dry milk powder

- teaspoons caraway seed

- 2 teaspoons active dry yeast

- 2/3 cup raisins

Directions:

- Place all ingredients (except for raisins) in the baking pan of the bread machine in the order recommended by the manufacturer.

- Place the baking pan in the bread machine and close the lid.

- Select Fruit Bread setting.

- Press the start button.

- Wait for the bread machine to beep before adding the raisins.

- Carefully remove the baking pan from the machine and then invert the bread loaf onto a wire rack to cool completely before slicing.

- With a sharp knife, cut the bread loaf into desired-sized slices and serve.

8. Mustard-Flavored Bread

Preparation Time: 25 minutes

Cooking Time: 2 - 3 hours Servings: 2½-pound loaf / 20 slices

Nutrition:

Total Carbs: 54g Fiber: 1g Protein: 10g Fat: 10g Calories: 340

Ingredients:

- 1¼ cups milk

- 3 tablespoons sunflower milk

- 3 tablespoons sour cream

- 2 tablespoons dry mustard

- 1 whole egg, beaten

- ½ sachet sugar vanilla

- 4 cups flour

- 1 teaspoon dry yeast

- 2 tablespoons sugar

- 2 teaspoon salt

Directions:

- Take out the bread maker's bucket and pour in milk and sunflower oil; stir and then add sour cream and beaten egg.

- Add flour, salt, sugar, mustard powder, vanilla sugar, and mix well.

- Make a small groove in the flour and sprinkle the yeast.

- Transfer the bucket to your bread maker and cover.

- Set the program of your bread machine to Basic/White Bread and set crust type to Medium.

- Press START.

- Wait until the cycle completes.

- Once the loaf is ready, take the bucket out and let the loaf cool for 5 minutes.

- Gently shake the bucket to remove the loaf. Transfer to a cooling rack, slice, and serve.

9. All-Purpose White Bread

Preparation Time: 25 minutes

Cooking Time: 2 - 3 hours Servings: 1-pound loaf / 8 slices

Nutrition:

Total Carbs: 27g Fiber: 2g Protein: 44 Fat: 2g Calories: 140

Ingredients:

- ¾ cup water at 80 degrees F

- 1 tablespoon melted butter, cooled

- 1 tablespoon sugar

- ¾ teaspoon salt

- 2 tablespoons skim milk powder

- 2 cups white bread flour

- ¾ teaspoon instant yeast

Directions:

- Add all of the ingredients to your bread machine, carefully following the instructions of the manufacturer.

- Set the program of your bread machine to Basic/White Bread and set crust type to Medium.

- Press START.

- Wait until the cycle completes.

- Once the loaf is ready, take the bucket out and let the loaf cool for 5 minutes.

- Gently shake the bucket to remove the loaf.

- Put to a cooling rack, slice, and serve.

10.   Ciabatta Bread

Preparation time: 20 minutes

Cooking Time: 1 hour

Servings: 24

Nutrition:

Calories 68 Total Fat 0.8 g Saturated Fat 0.1 g Cholesterol 0 mg Sodium 148 mg

Total Carbs 13.2 g Fiber 0.5 g Sugar 0.2 g Protein 1.9 g

Ingredients:

- 1½ cups water
- 1½ teaspoons salt
- 1 teaspoon white sugar
- 1 tablespoon olive oil
- 3¼ cups bread flour
- 1½ teaspoons bread machine yeast

Directions:

- Place all ingredients in the baking pan of the bread machine in the order recommended by the manufacturer.
- Place the baking pan in the bread machine and close the lid.
- Select Dough cycle.
- Press the start button.

- After the Dough cycle completes, remove the dough from the bread pan and place onto a generously floured surface.

- With a greased plastic wrap, cover the dough for 15 minutes.

- Line 2 baking sheets with parchment paper.

- Divide the dough into 2 portions and then shape each into a 3x14-inch oval.

- Place 1 bread oval onto each prepared baking sheet and dust with flour lightly.

- With plastic wrap, cover each baking sheet and set aside in a warm place for 45 minutes or until doubled in size.

- Preheat your oven to 425°F.

- Arrange the rack in the middle of the oven.

- Brush each loaf with water and bake for 25–30 minutes or until a wooden skewer inserted in the center comes out clean.

- Remove the loaf pans from the oven and place them onto a wire rack to cool for about 10 minutes.

- Now, invert each bread loaf onto the wire rack and coat with melted butter

- With a sharp knife, cut each bread loaf into desired-sized slices and serve.

Chapter 7: Cheese And Vegetable Bread Recipes

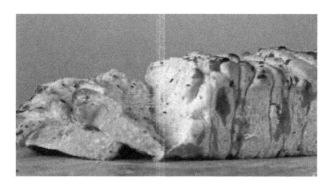

11.   Cracked Black Pepper Bread

Preparation time: 15 minutes

Cooking time: 3 hours

Servings: 16

Nutrition:

Calories: 152 kcal; Fat: 3.34 g; Carbohydrates: 26.24 g; Protein: 4.03 g; Sugar: 1.57 g

Ingredients:

- 4 cups of bread flour

- 1½ cups of water

- ¼ cup of Parmesan cheese, grated

- 3 tablespoons of sugar

- 3 tablespoons of chives, minced

- 3 tablespoons of olive oil

- 2 garlic cloves, crushed

- 2½ teaspoons of active dry yeast

- 2 teaspoons of salt

- 1 teaspoon of cracked black pepper

- 1 teaspoon of garlic powder

- 1 teaspoon of dried basil

Directions:

- Add all the ingredients to your bread machine pan according to the order suggested by the manufacturer.

- Select basic bread setting and press start.

12.   Zucchini Bread

Preparation time: 10 minutes

Cooking time: 2 hours

Servings: 16

Nutrition:

Calories: 115 kcal; Fat: 6.26 g; Carbohydrates: 13.02 g; Protein: 1.82 g; Sugar: 3.58 g

Ingredients:

- 1½ cups of unbleached all-purpose flour
- 1/3 cup of vegetable oil
- 1/3 cup of raisins
- 1/3 cup of packed brown sugar
- 1/3 cup of walnuts, chopped
- ¾ cup of zucchini, shredded
- large eggs
- tablespoons of granulated sugar
- ½ teaspoon of baking soda
- ½ teaspoon of baking powder
- ¼ teaspoon of ground allspice
- ¾ teaspoon of ground cinnamon
- ¾ teaspoon of salt

Directions:

- Add all the ingredients to your bread machine pan according to the order suggested by the manufacturer.

- Select quick bread or cake cycle and press start.

13.   Tomato Loaf

Preparation time: 10 minutes

Cooking time: 3 hours

Servings: 16

Nutrition:

Calories: 130 kcal; Fat: 2.95 g; Carbohydrates: 22.46 g; Protein: 4.01 g; Sugar: 1.56 g

Ingredients:

- 2 cups of all-purpose flour

- 1 cup of sour cream

- ½ cup of semolina flour or cornmeal

- ½ cup of whole wheat flour

- ½ cup of pitted black olives, well-drained, optional

- 1 6-ounce can of tomato paste

- 1 large egg

- 2½ teaspoons of instant yeast

- 1 teaspoon of dried basil

- 1 teaspoon of olive oil

- 1 teaspoon of white pepper

- 1 teaspoon sugar

- 1 teaspoon garlic powder

- ½-1 teaspoon of salt

Directions:

- Add all the ingredients to your bread machine pan according to the order suggested by the manufacturer.

- Select a quick bake cycle and press start.

14.   Butternut Squash Bread

Preparation time: 15 minutes

Cooking time: 3 hours

Servings: 18

Nutrition:

Calories: 239 kcal; Fat: 9.26 g; Carbohydrates: 34.95 g; Protein: 4.62 g; Sugar: 15.07 g

Ingredients:

- 3 1/3 cups all-purpose flour

- 2 2/3 cups white sugar

- 2 cups butternut squash, pureed and cooked

- 2/3 cup butter or shortening

- 2/3 cup water

- 4 eggs

- 2 teaspoons baking soda

- 2 teaspoons baking powder

- 1½ teaspoons salt

- 1 teaspoon ground cinnamon

- 1 teaspoon ground cloves

  Directions: Add all the ingredients to your bread machine pan according to the order suggested by the manufacturer.Select white or cake bread setting and press start.

15. Potato Bread

Preparation time: 5 minutes

Cooking time: 4 hours

Servings: 16

Nutrition:

Calories: 149 kcal; Fat: 2.85 g; Carbohydrates: 27.27 g; Protein: 3.5 g; Sugar: 1.57 g;

Ingredients:

- 3 cups of bread flour
- 1¼ cups of water
- 3 tablespoons of vegetable oil
- 2 tablespoons of potato flakes, mashed
- 7½ teaspoons of sugar
- 1½ teaspoons of active dry yeast
- 1 teaspoon of salt

Directions:

- Add all the Ingredients to your bread machine pan according to the order suggested by the manufacturer.
- Select basic bread setting and press start.

16.   Italian Herb Cheese Bread

Preparation time: 10 minutes

Cook time: 3 hours

Serves: 10

Nutrition:

Calories 247, Carbs 32.3g, Fat 9.4g, Protein 8g

Ingredients:

- Yeast – 1 ½ tbsp.

- Italian herb seasoning – 1 tbsp.

- Brown sugar – 2 tbsps.

- Cheddar cheese – 1 cup., shredded

- Bread flour – 3 cups.

- Butter – 4 tbsps.

- Warm milk – 1 ¼ cups.

- Salt – 2 tsps.

Directions:

- Add milk into the bread pan. Add remaining ingredients except for yeast to the bread pan. Make a small hole into the flour with your finger and add yeast to the hole. Make sure yeast will not be mixed with any liquids. Select basic setting, then select light crust and start. Once the loaf is done, remove the loaf pan from the machine. Allow it to cool for 10 minutes. Slice and serve.

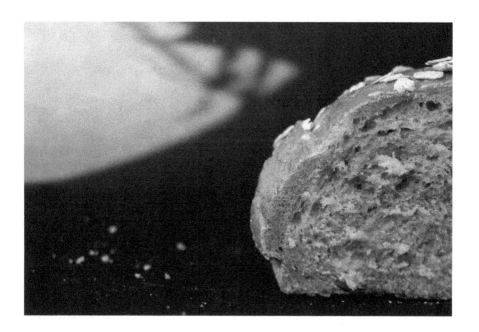

Chapter 8: Grain, Whole Wheat, Nuts And Seeds Bread Recipes

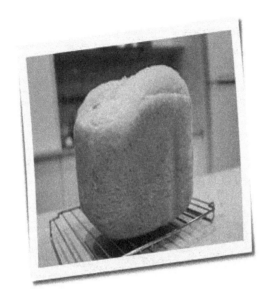

17.   Sesame Seeds & Onion Bread

Preparation Time: 30 minutes

Cooking Time: 2 - 3 hours Servings: 2½-pound loaf / 20 slices

Nutrition:

Total Carbs: 48g Fiber: 2g Protein: 10g Fat: 5g Calories: 277

Ingredients:

- ¾ cup water
- 3⅔ cups flour

- ¾ cup cottage cheese

- 2 tablespoons soft butter

- 2 tablespoons sugar

- 1½ teaspoons salt

- 1½ tablespoons sesame seeds

- 2 tablespoons dried onion

- 1¼ teaspoons dry yeast

Directions:

- Add all of the ingredients to your bread machine, carefully following the instructions of the manufacturer.

- Set the program of your bread machine to Basic/White Bread and set crust type to Medium.

- Press START.

- Wait until the cycle completes.

- Once the loaf is ready, take the bucket out and let the loaf cool for 5 minutes.

- Gently shake the bucket to remove the loaf.

- Transfer to a cooling rack, slice, and serve.

18. Caramel Apple Pecan Loaf

Preparation Time: 30 minutes

Cooking Time: 3 hours 50 minutes

Servings: 1-pound loaf / 8 slices

Nutrition:

Total Carbs: 32g Fiber: 2g Protein: 4g Fat: 5g Calories: 185

Ingredients:

- 1 cup water
- 2 tablespoons butter
- 3 cups bread flour
- ¼ cup packed brown sugar
- ¾ teaspoon ground cinnamon
- 1 teaspoon salt
- 2 teaspoons quick yeast
- ½ cup apple, chopped
- ⅓ cup coarsely chopped pecans, toasted

Directions:

- Add all of the ingredients to your bread machine (except apples and pecans), carefully following the instructions of the manufacturer.
- Set the program of your bread machine to Basic/White Bread and set crust type to Medium.

- Press START.

- Once the bread maker beeps, add pecans and apples.

- Wait until the cycle completes.

- Once the loaf is ready, take the bucket out and let the loaf cool for 5 minutes.

- Gently shake the bucket to remove the loaf.

- Transfer to a cooling rack, slice, and serve.

19. Orange Walnut Candied Loaf

Preparation Time: 30 minutes

Cooking Time: 24 hours

Servings: 1½-pound loaf / 12 slices

Nutrition:

Total Carbs: 82g Fiber: 1g Protein: 12g Fat: 7g Calories: 437

Ingredients:

- ½ cup warm whey
- 1 tablespoon bread machine yeast
- 4 tablespoons sugar
- 2 orange juice
- 4 cups flour
- 1 teaspoon salt
- 1½ tablespoons salt
- 3 teaspoons orange zest
- ⅓ teaspoon vanilla
- 3 tablespoons (walnut + almonds)
- ½ cup candied fruit

Directions:

- Add all of the ingredients to your bread machine, carefully following the instructions of the manufacturer.

- Set the program of your bread machine to Basic/White Bread and set crust type to Medium.

- Press START.

- Wait until the cycle completes.

- Once the loaf is ready, take the bucket out and let the loaf cool for 5 minutes.

- Gently shake the bucket to remove the loaf. Transfer to a cooling rack, slice, and serve

20. Awesome Multigrain Bread

Preparation Time: 30 minutes

Cooking Time: 2 - 3 hours Servings: 1-pound loaf / 8 slices

Nutrition:

Total Carbs: 27g Fiber: 2g Protein: 4g Fat: 2g Calories: 145

Ingredients:

- ¾ cup water at 80 degrees F

- 1 tablespoon melted butter

- ½ tablespoon honey

- ½ teaspoon salt

- ¾ cup multigrain flour

- 1⅓ cups white bread flour

Directions:

- Add all of the ingredients to your bread machine, carefully following the instructions of the manufacturer. Set the program of your bread machine to Basic/White Bread and set crust type to Medium.Press START.Wait until the cycle completes.

- Once the loaf is ready, take the bucket out and let the loaf cool for 5 minutes.

- Gently shake the bucket to remove the loaf.

- Transfer to a cooling rack, slice, and serve.

21. Sunflower Seeds & Oatmeal Bread

Preparation Time: 30 minutes

Cooking Time: 3 - 4 hours Servings: 1-pound loaf / 8 slices

Nutrition:

Total Carbs: 36g Fiber: 1g Protein: 6g Fat: 5g Calories: 200

Ingredients:

- 1 cup water
- ¼ cup honey
- 2 tablespoons butter
- 3 cups bread flour
- ½ cup quick-cooking oats
- 2 tablespoons dry milk
- 1¼ teaspoons salt
- 2¼ teaspoons bread machine yeast
- ½ cup sunflower seeds

Directions:

- Add all of the ingredients to your bread machine, carefully following the instructions of the manufacturer (except seeds.)
- Set the program of your bread machine to Basic/White Bread and set crust type to Light.
- Press START.

- Once the machine beeps, add seeds.

- Wait until the cycle completes.

- Once the loaf is ready, take the bucket out and let the loaf cool for 5 minutes.

- Gently shake the bucket to remove the loaf.

- Transfer to a cooling rack, slice, and serve.

22.   Whole Wheat Raisin Bread

Preparation time: 10 minutes

Cook time: 2 hours

Serves: 10

Nutrition:

Calories 290 Carbs 53.1g Fat 6.2g Protein 6.8g

Ingredients:

- Whole wheat flour – 3 ½ cups Dry yeast – 2 tsps.

- Eggs – 2, lightly beaten

- Butter – ¼ cup, softened

- Water – ¾ cup Milk – 1/3 cup Salt – 1 tsp.

- Sugar – 1/3 cup

- Cinnamon – 4 tsps.

- Raisins – 1 cup

Directions:

- Add water, milk, butter, and eggs to the bread pan. Add remaining ingredients except for yeast to the bread pan. Make a small hole into the flour with your finger and add yeast to the hole. Make sure yeast will not be mixed with any liquids. Select whole wheat setting, then select light/medium crust and start. Once the loaf is done, remove the loaf pan from the machine. Allow it to cool for 10 minutes. Slice and serve.

Chapter 9: Sweet Bread Recipes

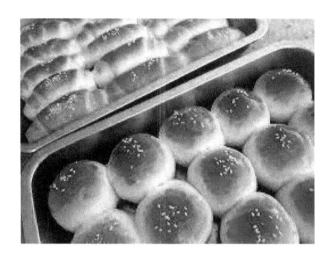

23.　Black Forest Loaf

Preparation Time: 20 minutes

Cooking Time: 3 hours

Servings: 2 ounces (56.7g)

Nutrition:

Calories: 136 | Carbohydrates: 27g Fat: 2g | Protein: 3g

Ingredients:

Dry Ingredients

- 1 ½ cups bread flour

- 1 cup whole wheat flour

- 1 cup rye flour

- 3 tablespoons cocoa

- 1 tablespoon caraway seeds

- 2 teaspoons yeast

- 1 ½ teaspoons salt

Wet Ingredients

- 1 ¼ cups water

- 1/3 cup molasses

- 1 ½ tablespoon canola oil

Directions:

- Combine the ingredients in the bread pan by putting the wet ingredients first, followed by the dry ones.

- Press the "Normal" or "Basic" mode and light crust color setting of the bread machine.

- After the cycles are completed, take out the bread from the machine.

- Cooldown and then slice the bread.

24. Cream of Orange Bread

Preparation Time: 20 minutes

Cooking Time: 2.5 to 3 hours

Servings: 2 ounces (56.7g)

Nutrition:

Calories: 190 | Carbohydrates: 30g Fat: 6g | Protein: 4g

Ingredients:

Dry Ingredients

- 2 cups rice flour

- ¾ cup potato flour

- 3 tablespoons sugar

- 2 tablespoons orange zest, minced

- 1 tablespoon xanthan gum

- ¼ teaspoons active dry yeast

- 1 teaspoon lemon zest, minced

- 1 teaspoon salt

- ¼ teaspoon cardamom

Wet Ingredients

- 3 eggs

- ¾ cup milk, half-and-half

- ¾ cup water

- 3 tablespoons vegetable oil

Directions:

- Add first the wet ingredients into the bread pan, then the dry ingredients.

- Set the bread machine to "Basic," "Normal," or "White" mode.

- Allow the machine to finish the mixing and baking cycles.

- Take out the pan from the machine.

- Wait for 10 minutes before transferring the bread to a wire rack.

- When the bread has completely cooled down, slice it and serve.

25. Tomato Bread

Preparation Time: 1o minutes

Cooking Time: 2 hours

Servings: 2 ounces (56.7g)

Nutrition:

Calories: 103 | Carbohydrates: 18g Fat: 2g | Protein: 3g

Ingredients:

Dry Ingredients

- 2 ½ cups gluten-free self-rising flour
- 2 teaspoons sugar
- ½ teaspoon Italian seasoning
- ½ teaspoon salt
- ¼ teaspoon ground nutmeg

Wet Ingredients

- 1 egg
- ¼ cup milk
- 6 tablespoons tomato paste
- 2 teaspoons olive oil

Directions:

- Combine all ingredients by putting the wet ingredients first into the bread pan, followed by the dry ingredients.

- Press the "Basic" or "Normal" mode of the bread machine with a light crust color setting.

- Wait for the cycles to be completed.

- Remove the bread from the machine to cool down completely before slicing.

26. Banana-Walnut Quick Bread

Preparation Time: 20 minutes

Cooking Time: 1.5 hours Servings: 2 ounces (56.7g)

Nutrition:

Calories: 160 | Carbohydrates: 21g   Fat: 7g | Protein: 4g

Ingredients:

Dry Ingredients

- 2 very ripe bananas, mashed

- ¾ cup sugar

- 2/3 cup rice flour

- 2/3 cup bean flour

- ½ cup tapioca flour

- ½ cup walnuts, chopped

- ¼ cup cornstarch

- 1 teaspoon baking powder

- ½ teaspoon baking soda

Wet Ingredients

- 2 eggs

- 2 tablespoons vegetable oil

Directions:

- Combine all ingredients in the bread pan, starting with the wet ingredients followed by the dry ones.

- Turn on the bread machine with the "Quick" or "Cake" mode on.

- Wait until the mixing and baking cycles are finished.

- Bring out the pan from the machine but keep the bread in the container for another 10 minutes.

- Transfer the bread to a wire rack.

- Slice the bread only when it has completely cooled down.

Chapter 10: Gluten-Free Bread Recipes

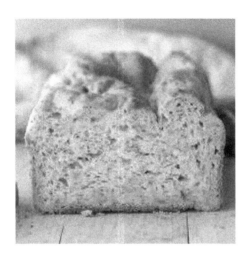

27. Paleo Bread

Preparation Time: 10 minutes

Cooking Time: 3 hours 15 minutes

Servings: 16

Nutrition:

Calories: 190, Fiber: 5.2 g, Fat: 10.3 g, Carbs: 20.4 g, Protein: 4.5 g.

Ingredients:

- 4 tablespoons chia seeds

- 1 tablespoon flax meal

- 3/4 cup, plus 1 tablespoon water

- 1/4 cup coconut oil

- 3 eggs, room temperature

- 1/2 cup almond milk

- 1 tablespoon honey

- 2 cups almond flour

- 1 1/4 cups tapioca flour

- 1/3 cup coconut flour

- 1 teaspoon salt

- 1/4 cup flax meal

- 2 teaspoons cream of tartar

- 1 teaspoon baking soda

- 2 teaspoons active dry yeast

Directions:

- Combine the chia seeds and tablespoon of flax meal in a mixing bowl; stir in the water, and set aside.

- Melt the coconut oil in a microwave-safe dish, and let it cool down to lukewarm.

- Whisk in the eggs, almond milk, and honey.

- Whisk in the chia seeds and flax meal gel and pour it into the beadmaker pan.

- Mix the cream of tartar and baking soda in the bowl and combine it with the other dry ingredients.

- Pour the dried ingredients into the bread machine.

- Make a little well on top and add the yeast.

- Start the machine on the Wheat cycle, light or medium crust color, and press Start.

- Remove to cool completely before slicing to serve.

28.   Sorghum Bread Recipe

Preparation Time: 5 minutes

Cooking Time: 3 hours

Servings: 12

Nutrition:

Calories: 169, Fiber: 2.5 g, Fat: 6.3 g, Carbs: 25.8 g, Protein: 3.3 g.

Ingredients:

- 1 1/2 cups sorghum flour
- 1 cup tapioca starch
- 1/2 cup brown or white sweet rice flour
- 1 teaspoon xanthan gum
- 1 teaspoon guar gum
- 1/2 teaspoon salt
- 3 tablespoons sugar
- 1/4 teaspoons instant yeast
- 2 eggs (room temperature, lightly beaten)
- 3 1/4 cup oil
- 1 1/2 teaspoons vinegar
- 3/4-1 cup milk (105 - 115°F)

Directions:

- Combine the dry ingredients in a mixing bowl, except for the yeast.

- Add the wet ingredients to the bread maker pan, then add the dry ingredients on top.

- Make a well in the center of the dry ingredients and add the yeast.

- Set to Basic bread cycle, light crust color, and press Start.

- Remove and lay on its side to cool on a wire rack before serving.

29.   Gluten-Free Potato Bread

Preparation Time: 5 minutes

Cooking Time: 3 hours

Servings: 12

Nutrition:

Calories: 232, Fiber: 6.3 g, Fat: 13.2 g, Carbs: 17.4 g, Protein: 10.4 g.

Ingredients:

- 1 medium russet potato, baked, or mashed leftovers
- 2 packets gluten-free quick yeast
- 3 tablespoons honey
- 3/4 cup warm almond milk
- 2 eggs, 1 egg white
- 3 2/3 cups almond flour
- 3/4 cup tapioca flour
- 1 teaspoon sea salt
- 1 teaspoon dried chives
- 1 tablespoon apple cider vinegar
- 1/4 cup olive oil

Directions:

- Combine all of the dry ingredients, except the yeast, in a large mixing bowl; set aside.

- Whisk together the milk, eggs, oil, apple cider, and honey in a separate mixing bowl.

- Pour the wet ingredients into the bread maker.

- Add the dry ingredients on top of the wet ingredients.

- Create a well in the dry ingredients and add the yeast.

- Set to Gluten-Free bread setting, light crust color, and press Start.

- Allow cooling completely before slicing.

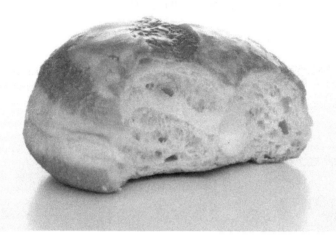

Chapter 11: Fruit And Sweet Bread Recipes

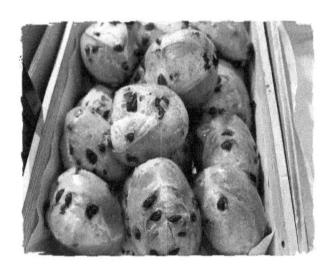

30. Cheese Pear Brioche

Preparation Time: 3 hours

Cooking Time: 45 minutes

Servings: 12 buns

Nutrition:

Calories 400, Fat 22.9 g, Carbohydrate 40 g, Fiber 1.9 g, Sugars 6.6 g, Protein 9.2 g

Ingredients:

For dough:

- 1/5 cup (50 ml) milk

- 5 eggs

- 1/3 cup (60 g, 2.4 oz.) sugar

- 3½ cups (500 g, 15¾ oz.) all-purpose flour

- 1½ teaspoon active dry yeast

- ½ teaspoon salt After beeping:

- 1 cup (225 g, 8 oz.) frozen butter, diced Filling:

- 1 pear

- 1 1/3 cup (170 g) cream cheese

For glaze

- 1 egg

Directions:

- Knead the dough in a bread machine. Take it out, wrap it with a kitchen film, and put it in the fridge overnight.

- Before you start cooking the buns, place the dough in a warm place for 1 hour.

- After that, cut the dough into 12 equal parts. Pinch a small piece of dough off each of the parts.

- Shape the big and small dough pieces into spheres. Place the large spheres in buttered cupcake baking cups and press your finger against the middle of their tops to make a little deepening.

- Peel and finely chop 1 pear and mix with soft cheese. Make a deepening in the large dough sphere, put the filling inside the deepening, and cover it up with the small sphere.

- Cover with a towel and leave for 1 hour to rest and rise.

- Preheat the oven to 350 degrees F (180 degrees C).

- Brush the surface of your brioches with a whipped egg.

- Bake in the preheated oven until golden brown for 15-20 minutes.

- Cool the brioche down on the grid.

- Serve and enjoy!

31.   Fruit Mini Buns

Preparation Time: 2 hours

Cooking Time: 45 minutes

Servings: 30 buns

Nutrition:

Calories 118, Fat 2.7 g, Carbohydrate 20.8 g, Fiber 0.7 g, Sugars 6.5 g, Protein 2.8 g,

Ingredients:

For dough:

- 1 cup (250 ml) milk

- ¼ cup (60 g, 2 oz.) butter

- 1 egg

- 1/3 cup (60 g, 2.4 oz.) sugar

- 3½ cups (500 g, 15¾ oz.) all-purpose flour

- 1½ teaspoon active dry yeast

- ½ teaspoon salt

For filling:

- 4 tablespoons apricot jam

- 4 tablespoons cherry jam

- Dried apricots, candied cherry

For garnish:

- 1 egg yolk

- ¼ cup (60 ml) milk

- 4 tablespoons ground almond

- 3 tablespoons colored sugar powdered sugar

Directions:

- Knead the dough in a bread machine. Let it rest and rise for 45 minutes.

- Divide the dough into 30 parts (approximately 30 g). Shape each piece of dough into a small round bun and place the buns on a baking sheet covered with oiled parchment paper. Leave for 15 minutes to rest and rise.

- Brush the buns' surface with milk-based egg wash. Sprinkle some of the buns with colored powdered sugar. Sprinkle the rest with chopped almonds.

- Make a little deepening on top of each bun. Fill it with your favorite major cover with dried apricots or candied cherries. Lightly flatten the buns.

- Cover with a kitchen towel and leave for another 30 minutes.

- Preheat the oven to 400 degrees F (200 degrees C).

- Bake in the preheated oven until golden brown for 8-10 minutes.

- Sprinkle with powdered sugar.

- Serve and enjoy!

32.   Brioche

Preparation Time: 3 hours

Cooking Time: 20 minutes

Servings: 12 buns

Nutrition:

Calories 344, Fat 18 g, Carbohydrate 37.9 g, Fiber 1.5 g, Sugars 5.5 g, Protein 8.1 g

Ingredients:

For dough:

- 1/5 cup (50 ml) milk

- 5 eggs

- 1/3 cup (60 g, 2.4 oz.) sugar

- 3½ cups (500 g, 15¾ oz.) all-purpose flour

- 1½ teaspoon active dry yeast

- ½ teaspoon salt After beeping

- 1 cup (225 g, 8 oz.) frozen butter, diced

For the glaze:

- 1 egg

Directions:

- Knead the dough in a bread machine. Take it out, wrap it with a kitchen film, and put it in the fridge overnight.

- Before you start cooking the buns, place the dough in a warm place for 1 hour.

- After that, cut the dough into 12 equal parts. Pinch a small piece of dough off each of the parts.

- Shape the big and small dough pieces into spheres. Place the large spheres in buttered cupcake baking cups and press your finger against the middle of their tops to make a little deepening.

- Put the small spheres inside the deepening's.

- Cover with a towel and leave for 1 hour to rest and rise.

- Preheat the oven to 350 degrees F (180 degrees C).

- Brush the surface of your brioches with a whipped egg.

- Bake in the preheated oven until golden brown for 15-20 minutes.

- Cool the brioche down on the grid.

- Serve and enjoy!

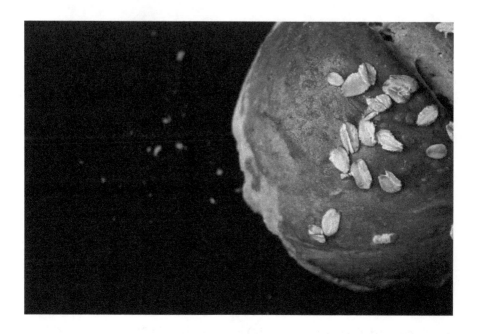

Chapter 12: Spice And Herb Bread Recipes

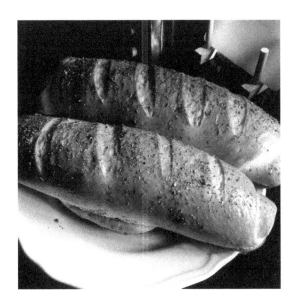

33.   Low-Carb Cauliflower Bread

Preparation Time: 20 minutes

Cooking Time: 45 minutes

Serving: 8

Nutrition:

398 Calories; 21g Fat; 4.7g Carbs; 44.2g Protein; 0 .5g Sugars

Ingredients:

- 2 cups almond flour

- 5 eggs

- ¼ cup psyllium husk

- 1 cup cauliflower rice

Directions:

- Preheat broiler to 350 °F.

- Line a portion skillet with material paper or coconut oil cooking shower. Put in a safe spot.

- In an enormous bowl or nourishment processor, blend the almond flour and psyllium husk.

- Beat in the eggs on high for as long as two minutes.

- Blend in the cauliflower rice and mix well.

- Empty the cauliflower blend into the portion skillet.

- Heat for as long as 55 minutes.

34.   Low Carb Flax Bread

Preparation Time: 10 minutes

Cooking Time: 24 minutes

Serving: 8

Nutrition:

Cal: 20, Carbs: 5g Fat: 13 g, Protein: 10g, Sugars: 5 g.

Ingredients:

- 200 g ground flax seeds

- ½ cup psyllium husk powder

- 1 tablespoon heating powder

- ½ cups soy protein separate

- ¼ cup granulated Stevia

- 2 teaspoons salt

- 7 enormous egg whites

- 1 enormous entire egg

- 3 tablespoons margarine

- ¾ cup water

Directions:

- Preheat broiler to 350 degrees F.

- Mix psyllium husk, heating powder, protein disengage, sugar, and salt together in a bowl.

- In a different bowl, blend egg, egg whites, margarine, and water together. On the off chance that you are including concentrates or syrups, include them here.

- Slowly add wet fixings to dry fixings and consolidate.

- Grease your bread dish with a spread or splash.

- Add the blend to the bread dish

- Bake 15-20 minutes until set.

35. Low-Carb Garlic & Herb Focaccia Bread

Preparation Time: 10 minutes

Cooking Time: 25 minutes

Serving: 7

Nutrition:

Cal: 80, Carbs: 16g, Fat: 7 g, Protein: 8g, Sugars: 10 g.

Ingredients:

- 1 cup Almond Flour

- ¼ cup Coconut Flour

- ½ teaspoon Xanthan Gum

- 1 teaspoon Garlic Powder

- 1 teaspoon Flaky Salt

- ½ teaspoon heating Soda

- ½ teaspoon heating Powder

Wet Ingredients

- 2 eggs

- 1 teaspoon Lemon Juice

- 2 teaspoon Olive oil + 2 teaspoons of Olive Oil to sprinkle Top with Italian Seasoning and TONS of flaky salt!

Directions:

- Heat broiler to 350 and line a preparing plate or 8-inch round dish with the material.

- Whisk together the dry fixings ensuring there are no knots.

- Beat the egg, lemon squeeze, and oil until joined.

- Mix the wet and the dry together, working rapidly, and scoop the mixture into your dish.

- Make sure not to blend the wet and dry until you are prepared to place the bread in the broiler on the grounds that the raising response starts once it is blended!!!

- 6 Smooth the top and edges with a spatula dunked in water (or your hands); at that point, utilize your finger to dimple the batter. Try not to be hesitant to dive deep into the dimples! Once more, a little water prevents it from staying.

- Bake secured for around 10 minutes. Sprinkle with Olive Oil heat for an extra 10-15 minutes revealing to dark-colored tenderly.

- Top with increasingly flaky salt, olive oil (discretionary), a scramble of Italian flavoring, and crisp basil. Let cool totally before cutting for an ideal surface.

36. Lemon & Rosemary Low Carb Shortbread

Preparation Time: 5 minutes

Cooking Time: 20 minutes

Serving: 6

Nutrition:

Cal: 100, Carbs: 2g, Fat: 10 g, Protein: 2g, Sugars: 4 g.

Ingredients:

- 6 tablespoons margarine

- 2 cups almond flour

- 1/3 cup granulated Splenda (or other granulated sugar)

- 1 tablespoon naturally ground lemon get-up-and-go

- 4 teaspoons crisp pressed lemon juice

- 1 teaspoon vanilla concentrate

- 2 teaspoons rosemary*

- ½ teaspoon preparing pop

- ½ teaspoon preparing powder

Directions:

- In a huge blending bowl, measure out 2 cups of almond flour, 1/2 tsp. Heating powder and 1/2 tsp. Preparing pop. Include 1/3 cup Splenda or other granulated sugar in the blend. Put in a safe spot.

- Zest your lemon with a Micro plane until you have 1 Tbsp. Lemon get-up-and-go. Squeeze a large portion of the lemon to get 4tsp lemon juice.

- In the microwave, liquefy 6 Tbsp. of margarine and afterward include 1 tsp. Vanilla concentrate.

- Transfer your almond flour and sugar to a little blending bowl. Put your spread, lemon get-up-and-go, lemon squeeze, and slashed rosemary into the now vacant huge blending bowl. Include your almond flour once more into the wet blend gradually, mixing as you go. Continue blending until all the almond flour is included back.

- Wrap the mixture firmly in cling wrap.

- Place the enveloped batter by the cooler for 30 minutes, or until hard.

- Preheat your stove to 350F, evacuate your batter, and unwrap it.

- Cut your batter in ~1/2" increases with a sharp blade. In the event that this blade isn't sharp, it will cause the batter to disintegrate. On the off chance that the mixture is as yet disintegrating, that implies it needs additional time in the cooler.

- Grease a treat sheet with SALTED margarine and spot your treats onto it.

Chapter 13: Loaf Bread Recipes

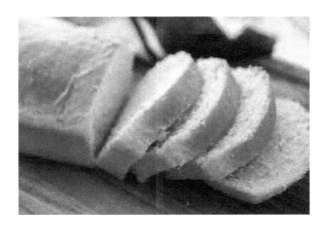

37. Morning Glory Loaf

Preparation time: 10 minutes

Cooking time: 3 hours 30 minutes

Servings: 12 slices/1.5lbs

Nutrition:

Calories: 116 Carbs: 20g Fat: 2g Protein:4g

Ingredients:

- Water, at room temperature 11/6 cups (278ml) 9fl oz.

- Light olive oil 2 tbsps. (30ml) 1 oz.

- Whole-meal bread flour 3 cups 13.7 oz. 390g

- Salt 1½ tbsp. 0.3 oz. 8.6g

- Soft brown sugar 1 tbsp. 0.44 oz. 13.6g

- Dried milk powder, skimmed 2 tbsps. 0.3 oz. 8.5g

- Muesli ½ cup

- Active dried yeast 2 tsps. 0.2 oz. 5.7g

Directions:

- Add olive oil and water, supported by half of the starch, to the machine.

- Now add the cinnamon, the starch, the powder of dry milk, the muesli, and the rest of the flour.

- Make a little dent or well in the top of the wheat and gently put the yeast into it so it doesn't touch any of the moisture.

- Close your machine's door, connect it to the wall and set it according to your machine's manual to the Whole Wheat configuration. Next, change the setting of the crust to your own personal liking.

- When cooked, remove the jar from the machine carefully and then take off the loaf, putting it to cool on a wire rack.

- Break the paddle after cooling and slice it with a sharpened bread knife.

38. Dark Bohemian European Bread

Preparation time: 7 minutes

Cooking time: 3 hours 20 minutes

Servings: 16 slices/2lbs

Nutrition:

Calories: 112 Carbs: 19g Fat: 3g Protein: 5g

Ingredients:

- Rye flour 11/2 cups 5.4 oz. 153g

- Bread flour 2 cups 9 oz. 254g

- Water at room temperature 11/4 cups (300 ml) 10fl oz.

- Olive oil 2 tbsps. (30ml) 1fl oz.

- Honey 3 tbsps. (44ml) 1.5fl oz.

- Caraway seeds (optional) 1 tsp.

- Fennel seeds (optional) ¼ tsp.

- Salt 1 tsp. 0.2 oz. 5.7g

- Active dried yeast 21/4 tbsps. 0.25 oz. 7g

Directions:

- Add ingredients to the bread machine according to the manufacturer's instructions. In mine, liquids always go first, so I start with water, olive oil, and honey.

- Mix the flours together so they're thoroughly combined. Then add half to your machine.

- Now add the caraway and fennel seeds if you like, as well as salt and remaining flour.

- Make a little well or dent in the top of the flour and carefully place the yeast into it, verifying it doesn't touch any of the liquid.

- Set the Basic/White setting, alter the crust setting to your own particular liking, and press START.

- Once cooked, carefully remove the bowl from the machine and remove the loaf before placing it on a wire rack to cool.

- Enjoy.

39. Carat Bread

Preparation time: 7 minutes

Cooking time: 3 hours Servings: 12 slices/1.5lbs

Nutrition:

Calories: 197 Carbs: 25g Fat: 5g Protein: 4g

Ingredients:

- Bread flour 2 cups 9 oz. 254g

- Whole meal bread flour 1 cup 4.6 oz. 130g Carrot juice 1 cup (240 ml) 8fl oz.

- Carrot, finely grated 1/2 cup

- Butter softened 2 tbsps. 1 oz. 30g

- Salt 1½ tbsp. 0.3 oz. 8.6g

- Brown sugar 1 tbsp. 0.44 oz. 13.6g

- Ground nutmeg (optional) 1½ tbsps.

- Bread machine yeast 2 tsps. 0.2 oz. 5.67g

Directions:

- Add ingredients to the bread machine according to the manufacturer's instructions. I usually start with liquids, then continue to add dry ingredients, except yeast.

- Make a little well or dent in the top of the flour and carefully place the yeast into it, making sure it avoids contact with any of the liquid.

- Mark the Basic/White loaf setting according to your machine's manual and Medium crust.

- Check the way the dough is kneading when five minutes elapse because the dough should turn into a smooth ball. You may need to add either one tbsp of liquid or one tbsp of flour, depending on the desired consistency.

- Once cooked, carefully remove the bowl from the machine and remove the loaf, placing it on a wire rack to cool.

- Once cool, remove the paddle; and for the very best results, slice with a serrated bread knife.

- Enjoy

Chapter 14: Breadstick, Crackers, Pizza, And Cookie Recipes

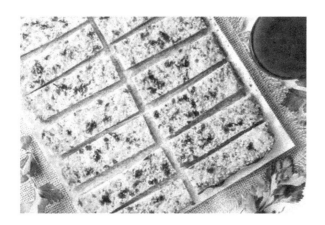

40.   Garlic Breadsticks

Preparation Time: 10 minutes

Cooking time: 20 minutes

Servings: 8

Nutrition:

Calories: 259.2, Fat: 24.7g, Carb: 6.3g, Protein: 7g

Ingredients:

For the garlic butter

- ¼ cup butter, softened

- 1 tsp. garlic powder

Other ingredients

- 2 cups almond flour

- ½ Tbsp. baking powder
- 1 Tbsp. Psyllium husk powder
- ¼ tsp. salt
- 3 Tbsp. butter, melted
- 1 egg
- ¼ cup boiling water

Directions:

- Preheat the oven to 400F. Line baking sheet with parchment paper.
- Beat the butter with garlic powder and set aside to use it for brushing.
- Combine the salt, psyllium husk powder, baking powder, and almond flour. Add the butter along with the egg and mix until well combined.
- Pour in the boiling water and mix until dough forms.
- Divide the dough into 8 equal pieces and roll them into breadsticks.
- Place in the baking sheet and bake for 15 minutes.
- Brush the breadsticks with garlic butter and bake for 5 minutes more.
- Serve.

41. Pumpkin Almond Cookies

Preparation Time: 10 minutes

Cooking time: 30 minutes

Servings: 12

Nutrition:

Calories: 315, Fat: 20g, Carb: 6g, Protein: 8.3g

Ingredients:

- 1 egg white

- 1 cup pumpkin puree

- 1 cup almond flour

- 1 cup almonds, ground

- 2 Tbsps. maple syrup, no sugar added

- ¼ cup coconut flakes

- ¼ cup lemon zest, grated

Directions:

- Combine flour, almonds, coconut flakes, and lemon zest.

- Whisk the egg white until foamy and gradually add maple syrup.

- Mix all ingredients together with pumpkin puree.

- Line a baking sheet with parchment paper and add the cookies by the spoonful.Bake at 300F for 30 minutes. Serve.

42. Cheese Spinach Crackers

Preparation Time: 15 minutes

Cooking time: 25 minutes

Servings: 16

Nutrition:

Calories: 126, Fat: 10.9g, Carb: 1.4g, Protein: 4.5g

Ingredients:

- 1 ½ cups almond flour

- 150g fresh spinach

- ½ cup flax meal

- ¼ cup coconut flour

- ½ tsp. ground cumin

- ¼ cup butter

- ½ cup parmesan cheese, grated

- ½ tsp. flaked chili peppers, dried

- ½ tsp. salt

Directions:

- Bring water to boil in a saucepan.

- Add spinach and cook for 1 minute.

- Add cooked spinach leaves into a cold-water bowl to stop the cooking process.

- Squeeze out the water from the spinach leaves and drain.

- Process the spinach in a food processor and process until a smooth consistency is reached.

- In the meantime, add almond flour, coconut flour, flax meal, cumin, chili flakes, salt, and parmesan cheese into the bowl and mix well.

- Add softened butter and spinach into the flour mixture and mix to combine well.

- Transfer dough into a refrigerator. Wrap in foil and keep for 1 hour.

- Preheat oven to 400F.

- Remove the foil wrapping and transfer the dough to a parchment paper-lined baking sheet.

- Top dough with second parchment paper piece and roll dough with a rolling pin until the dough is ¼ inch thick.

- Slice dough into 16 even pieces using a pizza cutter.

- Transfer baking sheet into the preheated oven and bake dough for 18 to 20 minutes.

- For a crunchier texture, adjust oven temperature to 260F and bake for 15 to 20 minutes more.

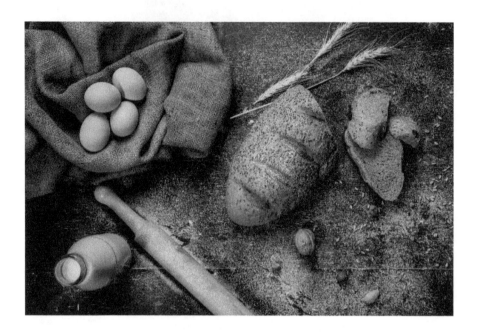

Chapter 15: Mixed Bread Recipes

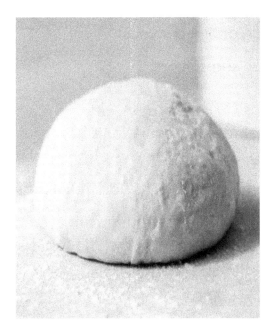

43.   Mustard Beer Bread

Preparation Time: 30 minutes Servings: 2 pounds / 20 slices

Cooking Time: 3 ½ hours

Nutrition:

Calories 284; Total Fat 3.3g; Carbohydrate 52.5g; Protein 7.9g

Ingredients:

- 4 cups (500 g) all-purpose flour

- 10 ounces (300 ml) dark beer

- 3 tablespoons granular mustard

- 1 teaspoon Dijon mustard

- 1 tablespoon butter, melted

- 1 tablespoon black molasses

- 1 teaspoon active dry yeast

- 1 teaspoon sea salt

Directions:

- Prepare all of the ingredients for your bread and measuring means (a cup, a spoon, kitchen scales).

- Carefully measure the ingredients into the pan.

- Place all of the ingredients into the bread bucket in the right order, following the manual for your bread machine.

- Close the cover.

- Select the program of your bread machine to BASIC and choose the crust color to MEDIUM.

- Press START.

- Wait until the program completes.

- When done, take the bucket out and let it cool for 5-10 minutes.

- Shake the loaf from the pan and let cool for 30 minutes on a cooling rack.

- Slice, serve and enjoy the taste of fragrant homemade bread.

44. Mediterranean Olive Bread

Preparation Time: 30 minutes

Cooking Time: 3½ hours

Servings: 2½ pounds / 24 slices

Nutrition:

Calories 299; Total Fat 7.7g; Carbohydrate 50.4g; Protein 6.8g

Ingredients:

- 4 cups bread flour

- 1 cup black/green olives, sliced

- 1 teaspoon active dry yeast

- 3 tablespoons extra virgin olive oil

- 1 tablespoon white sugar

- 1 ½ cups lukewarm water (80 degrees F)

- 1 ½ teaspoons sea salt

Directions:

- Prepare all of the ingredients for your bread and measuring means (a cup, a spoon, kitchen scales).

- Carefully measure the ingredients into the pan.

- Place all of the ingredients into the bread bucket in the right order, following the manual for your bread machine.

- Close the cover.

- Select the program of your bread machine to BASIC and choose the crust color to MEDIUM.

- Press START.

- Wait until the program completes.

- When done, take the bucket out and let it cool for 5-10 minutes.

- Shake the loaf from the pan and let cool for 30 minutes on a cooling rack.

- Slice, serve with some olives and enjoy the taste of fragrant homemade bread.

45.   Blue Cheese Onion Bread

Preparation Time: 30 minutes

Cooking Time: 3 hours 10 minutes

Servings: 1-pound loaf /
10 slices

Nutrition:

Calories 134; Total Fat 2.8g; Total Carbohydrate 21.9g;
Protein 4.9g

Ingredients:

- ¾ cup lukewarm water (80 degrees F)

- 1 whole egg

- 2 teaspoons butter, melted

- 3 tablespoons powdered skim milk

- 2 teaspoons white sugar

- ½ teaspoon kosher salt

- 1/3 cup blue cheese, crumbled

- 2 teaspoons dried onion flakes

- 2 cups all-purpose flour, sifted

- 3 tablespoons potato flakes, mashed

- ¾ teaspoons active dry yeast

Directions:

- Prepare all of the ingredients for your bread and measuring means (a cup, a spoon, kitchen scales).

- Carefully measure the ingredients into the pan.

- Place all of the ingredients into the bread bucket in the right order, following the manual for your bread machine.

- Close the cover.

- Select the program of your bread machine to BASIC and choose the crust color to MEDIUM.

- Press START.

- Wait until the program completes.

- When done, take the bucket out and let it cool for 5-10 minutes.

- Shake the loaf from the pan and let cool for 30 minutes on a cooling rack.

- Slice, serve with some olives and enjoy the taste of fragrant homemade bread.

46. Garlic Cream Cheese Bread

Preparation Time: 30 minutes

Cooking Time: 2 - 3 hours

Servings: 1 pound /8 slices

Nutrition:

Calories 179; Total Fat 6.2g; Total Carbohydrate 25.9g; Protein 4.9g

Ingredients:

- ⅓ cup lukewarm water (80 degrees F)

- ⅓ cup herb garlic cream cheese mix, at room temp

- 1 whole egg, beaten, at room temp

- 4 teaspoons butter, melted

- 1 tablespoon white sugar

- ⅔ teaspoon sea salt

- 2 cups all-purpose flour

- 1 teaspoon active dry yeast

Directions:

- Prepare all of the ingredients for your bread and measuring means (a cup, a spoon, kitchen scales).

- Carefully measure the ingredients into the pan.

- Place all of the ingredients into the bread bucket in the right order, following the manual for your bread machine.

- Close the cover.

- Select the program of your bread machine to BASIC and choose the crust color to MEDIUM.

- Press START.

- Wait until the program completes.

- When done, take the bucket out and let it cool for 5-10 minutes.

- Shake the loaf from the pan and let cool for 30 minutes on a cooling rack.

- Slice, serve and enjoy the taste of fragrant homemade bread.

47.   Fish Bell Pepper Bran Bread

Cooking Time: 3 hours Servings: 2 pounds / 20 slices

Nutrition:

Calories 208; Total Fat 3.8g; Carbohydrate 35.9g; Protein 7.2g

Ingredients:

- 2½ cups wheat flour

- ½ cup bran

- 1/3 cups lukewarm water

- 1½ teaspoons salt

- 1½ teaspoons brown sugar

- 1½ tablespoon mustard oil

- 1¼ teaspoons active dry yeast

- 2 teaspoons powdered milk

- 1 cup bell pepper, chopped

- ¾ cup smoked fish, chopped

- 1 onion, chopped and lightly fried

Directions:

- Prepare all of the ingredients for your bread and measuring means (a cup, a spoon, kitchen scales).

- Carefully measure the ingredients into the pan, except the vegetables and fish.

- Place all of the ingredients into the bread bucket in the right order, following the manual for your bread machine.

- Close the cover.

- Select the program of your bread machine to BASIC and choose the crust color to MEDIUM.

- Press START.

- After the signal, add all the additives.

- Wait until the program completes.

- When done, take the bucket out and let it cool for 5-10 minutes.

- Shake the loaf from the pan and let cool for 30 minutes on a cooling rack.

- Slice, serve and enjoy the taste of fragrant homemade bread.

48.   Rosemary Bread

Preparation Time: 30 minutes

Cooking Time: 2 - 3 hours Servings: 1-pound loaf / 8 slices

Nutrition:

Calories 175; Total Fat 6.2g; Carbohydrate 25.8g; Protein 4g

Ingredients:

- ¾ cup lukewarm water (80 degrees F)
- 1⅔ tablespoons melted butter, cooled
- 2 teaspoons white sugar
- 1 teaspoon kosher salt
- 1 tablespoon fresh rosemary, chopped
- 2 cups bread flour
- 1⅓ teaspoons instant yeast

Directions:

- Prepare all of the ingredients for your bread and measuring means (a cup, a spoon, kitchen scales).
- Carefully measure the ingredients into the pan, except the rosemary.
- Place all of the ingredients into the bread bucket in the right order, following the manual for your bread machine.
- Close the cover.

- Select the program of your bread machine to BASIC and choose the crust color to MEDIUM.

- Press START.

- After the signal, add the rosemary.

- Wait until the program completes.

- When done, take the bucket out and let it cool for 5-10 minutes.

- Shake the loaf from the pan and let cool for 30 minutes on a cooling rack.

- Slice, serve and enjoy the taste of fragrant homemade bread.

49.   Lavender Bread

Preparation Time: 30 minutes

Cooking Time: 3½ hours

Servings: 2 pounds / 20 slices

Nutrition:

Calories 226; Total Fat 1.1g; Carbohydrate 46.1g; Protein 7.5g

Ingredients:

- 1½ cups white wheat flour sifted

- 2 1/3 cups whole meal flour

- 1 teaspoon fresh yeast

- 1½ cups lukewarm water

- 1 teaspoon lavender

- 1½ tablespoon honey, liquid

- 1 teaspoon salt

Directions:

- Prepare all of the ingredients for your bread and measuring means (a cup, a spoon, kitchen scales).

- Carefully measure the ingredients into the pan, except the lavender.

- Place all of the ingredients into the bread bucket in the right order, following the manual for your bread machine.

- Close the cover.

- Select the program of your bread machine to BASIC and choose the crust color to MEDIUM.

- Press START.

- After the signal, add the lavender.

- Wait until the program completes.

- When done, take the bucket out and let it cool for 5-10 minutes.

- Shake the loaf from the pan and let cool for 30 minutes on a cooling rack.

- Slice, serve and enjoy the taste of fragrant homemade bread.

50. Salami Bread

Preparation Time: 30 minutes

Cooking Time: 3 hours 10 minutes

Servings: 1-pound loaf / 8 slices

Nutrition:

Calories 163; Total Fat 2.5g; Total Carbohydrate 28.6g; Protein 5.8g

Ingredients:

- ¾ cup lukewarm water (80 degrees F)

- 1/3 cup shredded mozzarella cheese

- 4 teaspoons sugar

- 2/3 teaspoon salt

- 2/3 teaspoon dried basil

- 1/3 teaspoon garlic powder

- 2 cups + 2 tablespoons wheat flour

- 1 teaspoon active dry yeast

- ½ cup finely diced hot salami

Directions:

- Prepare all of the ingredients for your bread and measuring means (a cup, a spoon, kitchen scales).

- Carefully measure the ingredients into the pan, except the salami.

- Place all of the ingredients into the bread bucket in the right order, following the manual for your bread machine.

- Close the cover.

- Select the program of your bread machine to BASIC and choose the crust color to LIGHT.

- Press START.

- After the signal, add the salami.

- Wait until the program completes.

- When done, take the bucket out and let it cool for 5-10 minutes.

- Shake the loaf from the pan and let cool for 30 minutes on a cooling rack.

- Slice, serve and enjoy the taste of fragrant homemade bread.

Conclusion:

Thanks for making it to the end. While using a bread machine can seem like an unnecessary step for others, without freshly home-baked bread, others do not imagine a life.

The freshly cooked, homemade bread can be enjoyed. Most bread manufacturers often provide a timer feature that enables you to schedule the baking period at a particular time. This is useful for breakfast anytime you need to get hot bread.

It is pretty straightforward to operate a bread machine. Some people claim it's untidy to bake bread at home, and usually, it's a challenging practice. With a bread machine, however, baking bread is easy. You just chose the perfect alternative and unwind - inside the bread machine, all the mixing, growing, and heating/baking phase is going on, which often makes it a zero mess process.

In the long term, it saves you a lot of money. You could be wrong if you believe that buying bread at a supermarket is cheap. It turns out that, particularly if you have any dietary restrictions, baking bread at home will save you cash in the long run.

CPSIA information can be obtained
at www.ICGtesting.com
Printed in the USA
BVHW011014150321
602551BV00001B/22